How to Banish Tiredness

For Better Sleep, Less Fatigue, Improved
Health and Energy

Alyson Rodgers

Disclaimer

Published by:
Alyson Rodgers and Random Technologies
4409 HOFFNER AVENUE, SUITE 347
Belle Isle, FL 32812

Subscribe to our newsletter for strategies to better
health, naturally!
www.naturesnaturalhealth.com/join

Table of Contents

INTRODUCTION

Whether you live in the "city that never sleeps" or a city where you discovered that saying applies to everywhere, chances are you have struggled with tiredness. Part of the problem is how busy we make ourselves—always on the go, never on a regular sleep schedule, running ourselves ragged until we finally collapse on our beds.

This is a major concern for health professionals, both mental and medical, and it should be concerning for us. If we are accustomed to being tired all the time, how will we know when our body is trying to warn us of an illness? How can doctors know that when we come in complaining of fatigue, we haven't been burning the midnight oil a little too long? How can we not understand how bad lack of sleep is for our bodies? These are all critical questions to ask about our often poor sleeping habits.

When you get into bad sleeping patterns, it is hard to get out of them. It creates a negative, repetitive cycle, which only multiplies its effects on your body.

Tiredness drives us all nuts, but it's a question of "has it driven us crazy enough to do the research and start solving the problems that underlie our lack of sleep". For example: many people do not realize how firmly tied to our eating habits our sleeping habits are. Our diet activities, our health oriented activities (do we take supplements, do we work out?), and our sleep routine all play into the quality of our sleep, and this book will walk you through why and what to do about it.

There is a lot that goes into giving you a good night's sleep. High amounts of sleep does not necessarily equal high quality of sleep. Quality of sleep is influenced by the night time routine, a good understanding of your personal needs, avoiding things like energy boosters (which throw off your schedule), and lowering stress levels, so you can actually relax. You can get 8 hours of sleep and still feel exhausted, or you can get 6 hours of sleep and feel fully rested.

If you follow the recommendations of this guide, you will be shocked to learn that setting yourself up for a good night's sleep actually sets you up for a good day. It goes beyond not needing your afternoon nap—you will be more alert, more focused, and perhaps better at remembering things. These benefits are available when you take care of your sleep cycle, which means if you aren't taking care of your sleep schedule, these are the things you're giving up.

This book is full of information geared towards helping you sleep better.

Stages of Sleep

Sleep can be your best friend if you use it correctly, or it can be your worst enemy if you're not. Poor quality sleep causes fatigue, memory issues, difficulty concentrating, and other issues. Understanding how your sleep works helps you understand how to make it better for you.

Research yielded five specifically unique stages of sleep. When researchers seek to study sleep, they connect willing subjects (using electrodes) to EEG technologies, which measures the electrical activity within the brain, to understand what is going on while we sleep.

You go through all five stages each night when you sleep, but you may be interrupted before you can reach stage five. This is related to the quality of sleep you are getting. Although all of the stages are important, stages four and five are the most important. This is because this is where deep, regenerative sleep truly occurs. The amount of sleep you get in these deeper stages influences how drowsy you will be the next day. It is an unfortunate reality that you actually spend the least amount of time in stages four and five.

Stage One:
(5 - 10 minutes in)
This is where you find yourself when you first close your eyes. The brain is slowing itself down progressively over the next 5 - 10 minutes. You're still somewhat alert, but you can feel yourself falling asleep. You can dream at this stage, or you can be in denial about sleeping. You usually aren't even aware

you're asleep at this stage.

Stage Two:
This is where your body starts to follow your brain's cues, and slows down—you even get cooler. It's harder to wake someone up from this stage, as it is slightly deeper than stage one, and their brain is actively engaged in sleep life.

Stage Three:
(30 - 45 minutes in)
This stage functions as the middle man between a shallow sleep state and a deep sleep state. Brain activity here is more regulated than in stage one or two, coming in consistently slow waves.

Stage Four:
This is where all of your most restful sleep occurs. Your body has completely let itself sink into a state of regeneration. It would be difficult to wake up a sleeper in this stage of sleep.

Stage Five:
(70 - 90 minutes after the beginning of the cycle)
This is the famous Rapid Eye Movement (REM) cycle, or rather, portion of the cycle known as REM. The body frequently reflects twitching and this could be consistent with brain activity. The brain is showing inconsistently short bursts of brain activity again, which may be a reflection of the hypothesis that most of our dreaming occurs at this stage.

Although somewhat speculative in research, this is the stage of sleep thought to be the most highly connected to our sense of focus and memory formation.

The typical cycle:
It is worth noting that although the stages are chronologically ordered, once you pass a stage, you can return to it. For example: a typical course of sleep is as follows: 1, 2, 3, 2, 3, 4, 5; and then reverses into 4, 3, 2, 1, and so on. As we progress through the stages, we get into progressively deeper sleep. Furthermore, the body consistently cycles through these stages several times per night (i.e., you go through this cycle more than once per night).

Another interesting fact involves the amount of time spent in stages four and five. In the first cycle, as mentioned above, it takes the longest amount of time to get into stages four and five, for the lowest amount of reward. As your body repeats the cycle throughout the night, you spend longer time in stage five, until your body prepares to wake up. As your body prepares itself to wake up, the only stages you go through are often one, two, and five.

So, how much sleep does your body actually want?
About two hours of deep sleep per night is the general recommendation. This can take hours to achieve. What happens if we mess up our sleep schedule? Our body temporarily becomes better at efficiently jumping into stage five of sleep.

Now that we have developed an adequate understanding of the stages of sleep, we can begin to identify and then counteract bad sleeping habits we already have.

Why does your body want it?

The body is negatively impacted by lack of sleep in several areas, from memory formation to reaction time and everything in-between. Common symptoms of exhaustion include: difficulty waking up, irritability, frequent accidents, clumsiness, dozing during the day, low quality performance, difficulty remembering things, poor decision making, and many more.

The first thing you may notice (depending on how tired you are) is you do not have a fast a reaction to things when you are tired. This is because your brain has not restored enough energy to work at its highest capacity. You can still process situations and information, but it will take significantly longer, and you will be less effective than if you were rested. This is related to all of the outward reactions to tiredness: increased chances of accidents, inhibition of motor skills, and spending longer on processing your information.

You also fail to commit things to memory (a lot more than you think) when you're tired. This is why your professors always cautioned you not to pull an all-nighter before the exam. You think you're getting a lot done, but the more tired you are, the less efficiently your brain absorbs the information you're studying. This relates to the functions of sleep.

Sleep helps us regenerate and reorganize information we have gained throughout the day. When we don't sleep, we don't get that reorganizing time; your brain doesn't get the chance to commit things to memory.

This does not only apply to your brain, it applies to your whole body. Your immune system's defenses are lowered when you are tired. Meaning, it's not a coincidence that we have the colloquial saying "sick and tired", it's a fact. When you are tired, you are more likely to get sick.

So, getting sleep doesn't just help you look better (bye-bye bags under the eyes), it helps you feel better and do better, too.

Let's look at some specific benefits of sleeping better.

Benefits of Quality Sleep

Beyond avoiding the negative side-effects of exhaustion, taking the steps to get a better night's sleep also has a lot of positive effects. Looking ahead to the future of a well-rested individual can be a powerful motivator to fixing your sleep schedule.

For starters, getting quality sleep helps you look better. The time you spend laying down helps battle the effects of gravity, decreasing your chances of wrinkles and reducing dark circles under the eyes. The time we spend sleeping also helps us regenerate, including shedding dead skin and growing new layers. The moral of the story: If you want to look younger, get some rest.

Further in the looks department, being tired has been linked to slimness. More accurately, research shows that hormones associated with appetite are also regulated by sleep. Also, people who are overweight do get significantly less sleep. So, want younger looking skin and slimmer bodies? Sleep.

There are also benefits for the heart that come from sleep. Losing sleep has been linked to several negative events, including high levels of cholesterol and blood pressure. The thing is, blood pressure and cholesterol are two of the best predictors of stroke and heart problems. Want to take care of your heart? Take care of your sleep.

The hormones associated with sleep are also associated with the body's level of cancer battling abilities. Daylight reduces these hormones and sleep increases them. You need to invest time in the quality of sleep, if you want to continue to bolster these positive hormones.

It's not only physical problems that sleep-induced hormones help prevent. When you are sleeping right, your stress levels are down, which means there is a lack of stress hormones pushed throughout your system. You're protected from stress more when you sleep well, than when you don't. You are similarly protected from depression. It's not a guarantee you won't suffer from these conditions, but it is a reduced likelihood.

Now that you know what sleep can do for your body, your mind, and your day, I assume you're convinced that it's a good idea to invest in sleeping better. Quality sleep means quality you.

Sleep Cycles

You may have guessed this by now, but in case you haven't, let me state the absolute bottom line about sleeping: this is not a guide about *how much sleep you are getting*. How many times have you stayed in bed all night (and some of the day), only to feel exhausted the next day? This is a guide about *what level* of sleep you are getting, as in: we have already explained the stages of sleep and I can guarantee that you are not getting stage 4 of sleep by dozing in and out of wakefulness.

A big problem that may seem obvious is we are creatures of habit. Our sleep cycles are as habitual as our coffee choices. We have to work to correct our sleep cycles, but once we put that work in, there will be consistent and predictably positive results.

Let's take a minute to recall how the sleep cycle works. Pretend sleeping is like a washing machine. A washing machine has several different cycles, each of which takes a different amount of time to complete. If you interrupt the wash cycle, you cannot expect your clothes to be rinsed; and when you reach the rinsing cycle, that doesn't mean there can't be a problem with the wash cycle's length. Your machine could easily be broken. What you want in terms of clean clothes is a machine that functions well.

This analogy is perfect for sleep. If you get interrupted in the middle of your sleep cycle, you cannot expect to get a good night's sleep. This is accomplished by teaching you tricks to optimize your personal sleep schedule.

Disclaimer: *This guide does not guarantee perfect sleep every night. It guarantees you the ability to set yourself up for a good night's sleep every night.*

Personal sleep cycles

Cycle 1	Cycle 2	Cycle 3	Cycle 4	Cycle 5	Cycle 6	Cycle 7
1.5 hours	3 hours	4.5 hours	6 hours	7.5 hours	9 hours	10.5 hours

Figure 1 is based on estimating a standard 1.5 hour sleep cycle

These figures are based on a 1.5 hour cycle and your cycle is individual to you. Once you figure out your sleep cycle, you need to optimize it by making sure you do not wake yourself in the middle of a cycle.

If your cycle finishes earlier than 9 hours, it will be better for you to wake up earlier than 9 hours. If you wake yourself between the cycles, you will be more tired than if you wake up later or earlier, to ensure getting up at the end of a full cycle. (i.e., 1.5 hours is better than 2).

One of the first steps to establish your personal sleep cycle is to keep a sleep journal to help fully analyze the effectiveness of your sleep.

Sleep Journals and Your Personal Sleep Cycle

Sleep journals log at least one week sleep, ideally beginning at the start of your week. Each entry needs to provide enough information for you to answer three specific questions: When did you go to bed? How long after going to bed did you fall asleep (approximately)? And when did you wake up (when did your eyes FIRST open)? If you have a significant other, or bed buddy, this can be a lot easier, as they can record the exact time you fell asleep and help you remember to write entries.

Make a note by your bed to remind yourself to be consistent with this!

Once you have logged a week's worth of information, you are ready to calculate your average. Add up the hours and divide the total by seven (for seven days), for both your total time spent sleeping and your time it takes to fall asleep.

Example in the table below: Time spent sleeping = 50.15 hours. Average time: 50.15/7 = 7.16 hour

The following table is a sample sleep log:

	MON	TUE	WED	THU	FRI	SAT	SUN
Bedtime	10:30 pm	11:00 pm	10:30 pm	11:15 pm	Midnight	1:00 am	10:30 pm
Time I fell asleep	10:50 pm	11:10 pm	10:45 pm	11:25 pm	12:25 am	1:10 am	11:00 pm
Time I woke up	6:05 am	6:15 pm	6:00 am	6:15 am	8:15 am	10:00 am	6:10 am
Time taken to fall asleep	20 mins	10 mins	15 mins	10 mins	25 mins	10 mins	30 mins
Time spent sleeping	6 hrs 15 mins	7 hrs 5 mins	6 hrs 15 mins	6 hrs 50 mins	7 hrs 50 mins	8 hrs 50 mins	7 hrs 10 mins

It is worth noting that during the week you record your sleep journal, you should not try to do anything different. We need to assess your natural sleep schedule, not your ideal best behaviour. This week does not have to be composed of consecutive nights (although, ideally, it would be). It can take several weeks to get seven days worth of uninterrupted sleep data.

Also, if at all possible, make sure you wake up and go to sleep naturally (no kids, alarm clocks, or animals). Nights that deviate from this (where something woke you up) must be discounted from the journal, as they do not reflect your body's needs accurately.

Using your sleep journal to establish your cycle
The average time it takes to complete a sleep cycle is between 60 - 120 minutes. Use this information in your sleep cycle calculations. Divide your sleep by potential cycle amounts, compare over time, and

alienate options as you go.

Example from the table above: On Friday, the person slept for 470 minutes (7 hours 50 minutes).
 If 4 cycles: 118 minutes, If 5 cycles: 94 minutes,
 If 6 cycles: 78 minutes

Five cycles seems most likely, but if you want to test this hypothesis, go to sleep (setting an alarm) for 118 minutes or 78 minutes, and record how you feel when you wake up: Rested, or groggy? Completed or interrupted?

This is one of those concepts that can seem complicated and intimidating, but is actually quite simple, and can help you get a drastically better night's sleep by figuring out your needs. Working in competition with your sleep cycle results in frustration and exhaustion. Cooperating with your sleep cycle needs will result in always waking up feeling rested, alert, and happier. Once you have assessed how much time it takes for you to complete a cycle, you can start building your sleep times around this (making sure you do not interrupt your own cycle).

If you plan efficiently, you may be able to do away with your alarm clock, as your body will naturally begin to wake up at a certain point after its cycles!

Developing Your Routine

Human beings are creatures of habit. We tend to enjoy the same type of juice we did when we were young, eat the same type of food, and do our hair similarly. This all adds up to one thing: you have a routine. Whether you are aware of it is another question entirely, but if you think about this, you will realize I am right.

So, what's my point? Our sleep is no exception. We all have a bedtime routine and an approximate bedtime (even without our parents telling us when it is).

This routine needs to be altered as we gain knowledge. Once you know what your required sleep needs are and you know what time you have to wake up, you know when your bedtime is. You should always try to protect your routine sleep needs, to ensure consistent and long lasting benefits that go with quality sleep.

Don't get me wrong, we all have exceptions, but the truth is you'll be far less tired if you stick to your routine on the weekend, as well as the weekday, than if you are constantly messing with your body. The stricter you are with yourself, the more firm your body will become in its rhythm, which in this case is a great thing: you developed a rhythm to help your body feel better!

This is the way you may come to not need an alarm clock, by setting a consistent amount of sleep for yourself. Help your brain help you.

Don't Hit Snooze!

We've all made friends with the snooze button at one time or another. You wake up to the alarm, mumble something about 10 minutes more, and hit the snooze button. *This could not be a worse idea*.

When you wake up desperate for "just a few more minutes", what your body is really saying is it was interrupted mid-cycle. We've already reviewed this, so you know that *every time* you close your eyes, you enter stage 1 of a new sleep cycle. This means "10 more minutes..." starts and interrupts another sleep cycle. Nobody's sleep cycle takes 10 minutes.

All snooze does is increases the amount of interrupted sleep cycles for you to contend with throughout the day. Not good folks, not good at all.

If, on the other hand, you force yourself out of bed the minute you wake up (please, trust me, I know what I'm saying), your brain will learn to back you up. What does this mean? It will develop to where your alertness is increased the moment you wake up.

This is within your power! This is not impossible! However, it is difficult and whoever said it wouldn't be was lying.

Causes of Tiredness (Outside of Cycles)

Sleep cycles are important. I cannot overstate this. However, sleep cycles are not the *only* important factor you need to take advantage of, if you want to get a great night's sleep.

Not all factors apply to all people, but knowing what factors can influence your sleep helps you identify which ones may be influencing you, specifically.

One major thing people don't think of when it comes to poor quality sleep is their diet. Some foods affect your energy levels—you can identify these foods and eat more, or avoid them accordingly. Additionally, sleeping habits are negatively linked to unhealthy weight patterns (over- or under-weight).

Another key factor is your physical activity level. Exercising helps the body regulate itself; if it's missing, then your sleep can suffer. This can be a bit of a vicious cycle in that, when you are very tired, you don't want to work out and when you don't work out, you continue to sleep poorly, at which point you're tired and don't want to work out, and so on.

Stimulant use also has a huge influence on the quality of sleep we get, whether illicit or not. Using stimulants either causes your energy levels to spike or fall. Even alcohol and nicotine affect energy levels, and thus quality of sleep. This is why some people can't drink coffee after six.

Sleeping problems obviously have an impact on the quality of sleep we get. Whether stress steps in and acts as the middle man, or sleep apnea disrupts our rest regularly, this is definitely a category.

Dehydration can also affect our sleep. This is because dehydration has numerous effects on the body, and tiredness is one of them. If you want to sleep well, you have to set your body up for it.

Each of these things can be overcome and/or dealt with. You have to determine which of these categories are impacting your sleep, so you can adjust accordingly.

In the following pages, we deal with recommendations that will help you get higher quality of sleep.

Circadian Rhythms and Melatonin

The term "circadian rhythm" refers to your body's natural regulation of sleep and wakefulness. Circadian rhythms are strongly influenced by light, which helps us sleep at night and stay awake during the day.

On top of light exposure, our body's hormones also regulate our urges of alertness and sleep. In particular, we will discuss melatonin and cortisol. Cortisol is a hormone associated with stress, but it also regulates alertness. Melatonin is typically released at night and is meant to regulate sleepiness. The two work together to keep your body in balance: melatonin starts at night and stops in the morning, then cortisol kicks in. However, they do not always function correctly.

In particular, not exposing yourself to enough light can cause higher-than-normal melatonin levels, which keeps you very tired. This means getting outside and keeping your rooms well-lit with natural light helps your body regulate tiredness.

It is worth noting that artificial lighting will not have the same effect as natural, since artificial has inferior effects. It is more important to open the curtains than to turn on a lamp. If you successfully expose yourself to enough natural light, your body's melatonin levels will be appropriately regulated and you will be more likely to get up right away. This is important for the reasons we talked about earlier.

The Effects of Stress on Your Sleep

Every one experiences stress. It's absolutely normal, but we don't have to take on unnecessary stress. There are plenty of ways you can avoid unnecessary stress and adequately manage stress levels of stress you cannot avoid.

One thing a lot of people struggle with is accepting that there are some things you cannot change. Accepting this reduces your worry about these things, which makes sense because worrying about something you can't change does nothing.

Focus your energy on the things you *can* change and looking optimistically at stressful situations, point out the good to yourself and focus on it, instead of the bad.

If there are situations you find stressful, prepare for them. Ensure that you have your support system in place. Work on rehearsing what will happen and practising healthy coping reactions. If all else fails, set up a new hobby that you can use to reward yourself, for handling stress in a healthy manner.

Tips for managing stress:
- Make a to-do list. A to-do list lets you know what you have to get done and what should be done first.
- Be realistic in personal expectations. Don't try to force yourself to be superhuman, because you can't be superhuman. You will only discourage yourself by setting unachievable goals.
- Associate with positive people in your life, who encourage your positive habits.

- Reduce your intake of potentially harmful substances, like nicotine and alcohol, or eliminate them from your life entirely.
- Accept that there are things you cannot change, no matter how hard you try – and *do not worry about them*
- Prepare yourself for situations you know you will find stressful

Tips for avoiding stress:
- Take things off of the to-do list. Do the things you can do, remove the things you can't or the things that can wait.
- Learn to not put tasks that aren't worth doing onto the to-do list. This means learning to say "no" to tasks you know you don't have time for and learning when enough is enough.
- Avoid stressful people. People who stress out frequently are stressors for you, unnecessary ones.
- Learn what stresses you out and either how to manage it or get rid of it.

These tips work together to ensure you have the ability to not be constantly stressed out. Stress keeps you from sleeping well, by keeping your body in a heightened state of alertness. Increased alertness disrupts our sleep throughout the night and makes it difficult to fall asleep, at all. This is significantly connected to the amount of sleep you get in the fifth stage.

This is why learning to deal with stress is so critical to help you sleep better.

Relax and End Tiredness

Stress directly and negatively correlates with the quality of your sleep. The more stressed you are, the less restful sleep you get. Thankfully, the opposite is also true: The more relaxed you are, the more quality sleep you will get. Since we already considered stress reduction methods, it is time to consider relaxation techniques.

There are several techniques you can use to ensure your body is relaxed. While some of them can take a significant amount of time to learn, knowing how to relax is well worth the effort.

Breathe
This may sound humorously obvious, but you'd be shocked by how often you aren't giving your body enough oxygen. So, take a minute and practice this technique:

Sit down in a quiet room, in a comfortable chair. Focus on feeling your feet flat on the floor and the relaxation that comes with your back, shoulders, and neck being fully supported.

Count slowly to four, while inhaling through your nose. Hold that breath for two seconds. Feel that breath filling your body. Then release that breath, slowly, while counting to six. Repeat these steps until you feel the relaxation flowing through you.

This technique is generally mastered by 10 minutes of practice a day and has been found to slow your heart rate, lower blood pressure, and release tension within your muscles. Once you have mastered this technique, you will be surprised at how natural it becomes to you, to the point that when you feel yourself getting stressed, you can practice it and instantly reap the relaxing rewards. This is not the only technique, however.

Let's talk about sighing; specifically, the Sigh Breath. Inhale slowly through your nose. Hold on, take a pause, and then breathe out through your nose. Don't blow it out. Breathe out slowly, as though regretful of your need to let the air go. As the air leaves, so does the tension within your body. Feel the tension leaving your head, your neck, now your shoulders, and so on. Take a second to enjoy that before taking your next breath.

As you breathe in again, focus your energy. What is going on? Focusing on slowly analyzing the situation around you can calm you down in the most extreme situations. Eventually, once mastered, this technique enables you to focus without being anxious about the situation at hand—no matter how terrible it may seem to other people.

This technique specifically focuses on releasing tension within the body and takes you out of an immediately stressful situation. It's especially handy because no quiet room is necessary, you simply breathe in and out, and feel the tension go with it.

Breathing techniques are quite popular. The way we breathe relates to our intake of oxygen, which relates to how hard our body has to work to keep itself running (the more oxygen you provide yourself, the less you have to work). The primary focus of each of these techniques is to fill your lungs with air and enjoy the feelings that a relaxed body produces.

Sit down

While sitting down, focus on relaxing your body. Focus on the way your feet are connecting with the floor. Feel how heavy and warm they are, and how that feeling is moving up your legs, slowly. Feel it crawl up your calves, into your knees and thighs. Breathe deep, help this feeling of relaxation spread throughout your body, relaxing yourself even further. Let your body get heavier and heavier as you sit, even your eyes as you slowly give in to the relaxed tiredness your body is experiencing.

Lay down

You may be accustomed to the idea of "having a lay down", but this is different, so please, pay attention. When we lay down, we often focus on the release of pressure on our backs; it feels good to be off our feet. This technique works a little more specifically.

Lay back (with your eyes closed), somewhere you feel comfortable. Wriggle your toes, then ease them in an upwards direction (towards your face) for ten solid seconds. Relax, take a ten second break, and repeat. Toes can be a great way to focus your relaxation, because they represent such a moveable point on your body and signify an area of the body that represents a lot of stress and pressure (your feet). Most people overlook them, but this is a great way to help you relax.

Visualization

Visualization is literally closing your eyes and focusing your mind on a place. When practiced, you can use visualization anywhere, but to start it should be done in a silent room, where you know no one will bother you. You can visualize any place at all, so long as that place represents relaxation to you. Let your mind take you there, exploring what there is to see and sensing every bit of the scene that you can. This is incredibly relaxing and can be done in blocks of five full scenes.

Example scenes: Imagine yourself on a beach, Imagine yourself in a forest, Imagine yourself on vacation, Imagine yourself atop a mountain

Remember, in each scene the point is to focus on the sights, smells, and feelings that each of the settings evoke in you. This is a very relaxing technique.

If you are struggling with these techniques, there are plenty of DVDs and CDs to teach you how to do it. Make sure you're listening to these things in a relaxing room, instead of while driving; you have to be okay with drifting off to sleep. Intense relaxation is not so conducive with high-pressure traffic.

Remember, the less stressed you are, the easier you'll relax. The more you relax, the better your sleep and isn't that everyone's goal?

Evening Routines

We have spoken extensively about how and why stress impacts our sleep, and how to combat these effects. Now, it's time to consider how our nightly routine impacts our time spent in bed.

Developing your evening routine aids the goal of setting yourself up for a good night's sleep. The more habitually you set up a routine, the more your brain will respond to that habit. The brain is a huge key in the quality of sleep that we get.

The focus of your night time routine should be what you do before bed. You need to make sure that this routine is as relaxed and consistent as possible. Somewhat intuitive, avoid stressful activities before bed. This means if you have a test you're "cramming" for, stop studying at least an hour before sleep time. If you hate scary movies, you should not be watching *Saw* before you go to sleep. Following these tips will help you fall asleep and sleep well.

A favourite pre-bedtime activity: Take a warm bath before you wind down for bed (at least an hour between bath time and bedtime). You can add bubbles, oils, or simply light some aromatherapy candles.

An example of a full routine would be: taking a bath, doing some reading with a warm cup of hot chocolate, and then drifting off to sleep.

Morning Routines

Why is getting out of bed in the morning so hard? A big part of it is what we do when we get out of bed. For most of us, we wake up at the last possible second to finish up extra work, get dressed, quickly brush our teeth, and run out the door (often forgetting our keys). What part of that process sounds fun or enticing to you? None of it does. It's no wonder you want to stay in bed all day. You can't get frustrated at red lights in bed, or forget where you put your car keys; sometimes, it feels like you can't even be running late, so long as you're in bed.

To further illustrate this point, consider how little trouble you probably have waking up Christmas morning. Why? Because you're excited about what's going to happen. You need to work on creating a morning routine that makes you happy to get out of bed. Whether it's picking up your favourite kind of bagel or making time to do yoga before work, motivate yourself!

We've already discussed the importance of getting straight out of bed when your alarm goes off, but who wants to run around and get the opportunity to be rushed? Nobody does. Thus, working on a healthy morning routine can help us get better quality sleep.

For most people, this means not getting up 2 minutes before you need to be out the door. Give yourself some time to enjoy a nice breakfast, kiss your significant other hello, or check the emails if you want. The morning can also be a great time to exercise, since increasing physical activity in your life is another great way to improve your body. Whatever it is that you enjoy doing, make sure you do some of it in the morning. It makes that climb out of bed seem all the less treacherous.

Food and Sleep

Diet is another area of life that has huge effects on how we sleep. A lot of people don't take this seriously, but I challenge you to try it: make sure you're eating well for a certain amount of time and see the effects for yourself. Diet is one part of keeping your body healthy and a healthy body is a rested body.

Why should we care about food and sleep?
To show you how food can impact your sleep schedule, let's focus on looking at what happens when unhealthy eating patterns take over and your body lacks the necessary fuels (vitamins) to keep going.

Anemia – An iron deficiency that results in extreme tiredness. Can be corrected temporarily with iron supplements, but eating right is the best way to get iron.

Vitamin deficiencies (example: Vitamin B deficiencies) – Vitamin deficiencies of any kind, but particularly those in the B group, cause extreme fatigue.

So what qualifies as "eating well"?
First, make sure you're eating. You should be eating regularly and you should be eating well. Interestingly enough, our three-meal-a-day standard may not be as effective as having five-to-seven smaller meals. This is because the bigger the meal, the more likely you'll take an after-meal nap, due to drowsiness—something that messes with your sleep schedule.

Second, make sure that on top of eating regularly, you are not eating within three hours of bedtime. Food is good for us, but it makes our body work, and at sleep time your body needs to be utterly relaxed. If you need a snack before bed, make it a light and healthy one. Eating does not help us rest, but eating well does help us sleep better when we sleep.

Foods to avoid near bedtime: ham, bacon, sausage, chocolate, and cheese.
Foods that increase alertness: Nuts, bananas, peanut butter, and green veggies.

In terms of specific meal requirements, make sure you're getting five portions of fruit and vegetables every day (this can work through fruit juice, as well), eat lean meats when possible, focus on good carbohydrates, and try to avoid sugars and fatty foods. These are all foods that either help you or hurt you. You need to make sure you're focused on eating foods that help you. Consult your local food guide for further specific guidelines.

If you aren't eating well, at least ensure you are getting all of your vitamins—whether through your meals or through supplements.

These recommendations are made because both people who are underweight and overweight have been shown to struggle with sleep. Correcting an unhealthy diet will help not only with your quality of sleep, but with any applicable weight issues.

These changes should not necessarily be made instantaneously, but they should be made. The reason I recommend you not do it all at once is because this increases the chances of returning to your old habits. You have developed an unhealthy eating pattern for years, so you can't expect to fix it in a day.

Does warm milk help?

We've all heard the old adage about drinking a glass of warm milk before bed, but does it work? Research has shown that warm milk does, in fact, help us sleep. This is related to what it does within the body. Milk's products turn to serotonin within the body, which, as we said earlier, is a well-established link with sleeping well.

Water and Sleep

Let's take a step back from the general category of diet and discuss one aspect: beverages. There are drinks you should avoid (that will be discussed later) and drinks you probably need more of. One such drink that belongs in the latter category is water.

Making sure you get enough water keeps your body hydrated, so it functions better. We look and feel better when we are properly hydrated. Our bodies are actually made of mostly water, so it's pretty important to drink, for energy. Drinking water is one of those tips I am happy to give in this guide, because I know it will bring results to your sleep and your life, as a whole.

The problem is most of us are not drinking enough water and we're paying the price in ways we don't often associate with drinking—our waists and our beds. Thirst is often confused with hunger. Hunger often results in eating something that's going to disrupt your sleep schedule. Drinking water prevents this problem (and others) entirely.

Do you know what "enough water" is? Eight glasses a day. This amount can vary individually, but the general recommendation is 8 glasses of water a day. Take a moment to assess how much water you're drinking and it's likely you'll find it's nowhere near enough.

It is worth noting that although we do get some water from other foods and drinks, there is no substitute for water itself. However, if you are struggling to get enough water, here are some helpful tips on increasing your water intake:

Simple ways to increase your water intake

- Always make water available to yourself.
  Whether this means putting some in your car, or constantly refilling a water bottle or mug you carry with you, ensure that water is always nearby. This will encourage consistent sipping, which will result in a higher water intake.

- Drink before you eat.
  This works in two ways: eating will remind you to drink and drinking before you eat will prevent you from potentially confusing thirst with hunger.

- Treat the taste buds with fruit.
  Some people complain about the taste of water. Beyond the obvious option of getting a filter, I recommend adding a slice of fruit (lemon or lime being the popular choices).
  (Helpful hint: Try freezing sliced fruit and dropping it into your drink like ice cubes!)

- Drink early and drink often.
  Try to drink right when you wake up, right before each meal, and a few glasses before you go to sleep. This encourages developing your water intake into a steady routine that will easily transition into a healthy habit for the future.

- Replace bad drinks with good ones
  Always drink water after caffeinated products, alcoholic products, and ultimately instead of these products, to counteract their effects. We will discuss these effects at length later, but for now believe me, they need counteracting.

It can also encourage a connection in your mind with water and thirst, instead of bad beverages and thirst, which can increase your water intake and decrease the intake of potentially harmful substances.

Signs you weren't previously drinking enough water

So, what's the best confirmation that you weren't getting enough water, before you tried all this? Trying all this and seeing how it makes you feel.

For a lot of people, the difference is relatively instant (within a few weeks). Decreased headaches, decreased tiredness, increased alertness, and even improved appearance can be among the outwardly obvious health benefits that appear. If these and your water drinking habits are new, the logical deduction is that you were not getting enough water before.

Water intoxication

I will leave you with one very important warning. While it is very important that you get enough water, it is a horrible idea to drink too much water at once. This can flood your organs, literally drowning them if you're not careful.

Putting it all Together: Food and Drink

Both dietary nutrition and water intake are absolutely critical to the quality of sleep you get. It is vital that you work with both of these bodily needs, to keep yourself prepped for a good night's rest.

When we rest, our body regenerates. This requires the right fuels, in the right amounts. When we fail to provide these fuels, the body does not work as well when it sleeps or when it's awake, leading to a lot of the dangers when you don't supply yourself with enough water, or the right food.

Lack of sufficient water supply can lead to increased blood clots, lack of alertness, headaches, dizziness, extreme hunger (which may actually be extreme thirst), and improper regulation of bodily toxins (less drinking, less trips to the toilet, more toxins stored up).

Lack of sufficient food can lead to fatigue, trouble concentrating, overeating, unhealthy weight issues, and much more.

Summary of advice
- Try to drink 8 glasses of water a day (using the tips above)
- Make sure you're getting 5 servings of fruits and veggies each day
- Eat regularly and eat well
- Don't eat within a few hours of going to bed, but if you must, keep it light

By following the advice here, you will get your best chance at optimizing your body for a good night's sleep.

Let's talk about some of the substances you need to avoid to do this.

Harmful Effects of Caffeine

A lot of us enjoy a regular cup of coffee in the morning, a coke with lunch, or a tea after dinner. What most of us don't realize, however, is this is a direct result of not sleeping the best we can. We need a pick-me-up because we feel lower-than-normal in energy levels.

The bigger problem is caffeinated drinks pick you up for a very short amount of time and in the long-term they prevent you from sleeping. It prevents you from sleeping by spiking your body's heart rate and breathing. So, your body gets very confused, not knowing what it's doing or if it's right or wrong, and your sleep will suffer as a result.

Interestingly, your mood also suffers. You can get headaches, suffer from increased irritability, and exhaustion when your caffeine levels decrease. Caffeine is also an addictive substance, which can multiply these symptoms. Not the least of which is: the more you force your body through these highs and lows, the more tired your adrenal glands (which produce adrenaline) become.

The summary: Caffeine is a band-aid for a low quality sleep problem. Caffeine is not the only stimulant, though.

Reducing caffeine, or even cutting it out altogether, is something highly recommended. This helps us optimize our sleep schedule and benefit our own health.

Special notes for caffeine and pregnancy

Research has shown, time and time again, there are significant effects on the fetus, including low birth weight and in some cases, miscarriage.

People often overlook caffeine as a pregnancy risk, especially when already eliminating nicotine and alcohol from their repertoire. This is very disturbing, given the findings, which should not be ignored.

Most recently, a study concluded that a mere 300mg of caffeine a day (three mugs of coffee, six cups of tea, eight chocolate bars [there is less caffeine in milk chocolate], and so on) was enough to link with risks like miscarriage and low birth weight. Low birth weight is associated with a host of long term medical issues for children. That child could suffer very seriously for your morning cup of coffee, so please indulge carefully.

If you are pregnant and trying to cut back, or cut out caffeine in your life, please see the tips listed for how to replace it carefully.

Common Foods and Medications Caffeine Content

Substance	Serving Size (volume or weight)	Caffeine Content (range)	Caffeine Content (typical)
Coffee			
Brewed/Drip	6 oz	77-150 mg	100 mg
Instant	6 oz	20-130 mg	70 mg
Espresso	1 oz	30-50 mg	40 mg
Decaffeinated	6 oz	2-9 mg	4 mg
Tea			
Brewed	6 oz	30-90 mg	40 mg
Instant	6 oz	10-35 mg	30 mg
Canned or Bottled	12 oz	8-32 mg	20 mg
Caffeinated Soft Drinks	12 oz	22-71 mg	40 mg
Caffeinated Water	16.9 oz	50-125 mg	100 mg
Cocoa/Hot Chocolate	6 oz	2-10 mg	7 mg
Chocolate Milk	6 oz	2-7 mg	4 mg
Coffee Ice Cream or Yogurt	1 cup (8oz)	8-85 mg	50 mg
Chocolate Bar			
Milk Chocolate	1.5 oz	2-10 mg	10 mg
Dark Chocolate	1.5 oz	5-35 mg	30 mg
Caffeinated Gum	1 stick	50 mg	50 mg
Caffeine-Containing OTC Products			
Analgesics	2 tablets	64-130 mg	64 or 130 mg
Stimulants	1 tablet	75-350 mg	100 or 200mg
Weight-loss products	2-3 tablets	80-200 mg	80-200 mg
Sports Nutrition	2 tablets	200 mg	200 mg

Taken from: www.caffeinedependence.org/
caffeine_dependence.html

Caffeine as an Addictive Substance

Caffeine is a huge part of our culture, present in many different types of products. Many people have heard caffeine is bad for you, but what everyone doesn't know is how addictive it is. Some people are likely laughing right now, not taking this seriously, but the following paragraphs will outline how serious caffeine addiction can be.

Caffeine faces a surprising lack of regulations governing it, especially considering it is formally classed as a psychoactive substance. While it normally functions as a relatively harmless substance, indulging excessively leads to negative consequences on the body, including issues with increased heart rate, dehydration, and restlessness. The amount of caffeine it takes to produce these effects varies between individuals. In extreme situations, some people become addicted to caffeine.

Becoming addicted creates a need for an extremely unhealthy amount of caffeine, which incurs all of the negative benefits from above, plus the possibility of withdrawal, if the individual ever lacks access to adequate amounts. In the event of developing a caffeine addiction, it is recommended that you carefully and gradually cut back on caffeine. It must be a gradual cutback, to avoid withdrawal.

It should also be noted that those addicted to caffeine have increased risk for caffeine induced intoxication and even hallucinations. Warning signs of addiction include heart palpitations, headaches, and irritability.

This information should make you strongly consider moderating your caffeine consumption. If you do not already drink an appropriate amount, consider either cutting back or entirely eliminating caffeine from your diet.

The Benefits of Caffeine

We've taken a pretty harsh look at caffeine, but the truth is it's not *entirely* bad for you. Let's take a look at some of its benefits, so you can see the entire picture.

One of the paradox-inducing effects of caffeine is it increases the level of cortisol. We have discussed cortisol as a stress hormone and it is, but it also can be good for the body *in moderation*. Cortisol puts the body into fight or flight mode. While this is bad for you long-term, in the short-term it means many positive things, most importantly of which is it makes your body run efficiently.

The metabolism speeds up when the body is in this mode and this means that fat will be broken down with increasing efficiency, but only when you exercise as well as drink caffeine.

All of the problems (increased heart disease and stroke risk, poor sleeping quality, and so on) start when you have too much caffeine. However, it is possible to balance some of the positive and negative effects. The key is not to ingest too much caffeine, so reducing your intake (if not cutting it out altogether), is still entirely a worthy option.

It's your job to make an informed decision. Some people think caffeine is too dangerous to toy with, while others are fine with it. Which group you fall into will depend on how you weigh the positives and negatives of caffeine that we have so carefully laid out.

Quitting Caffeine

Cutting caffeine out of your life is not the easiest decision. Caffeine is often built directly into our morning ritual and certainly into our social ones. It's common practice to ask your friends to "go for a cup of coffee" or "not speak to you 'til you've had your morning coffee". This makes it a very hard habit to break. Hard to break is not impossible to break, however, and the following paragraphs outline helpful tips for quitting caffeine.

The first step is to alter your existing routine. Instead of having a cup of coffee, perhaps mixing half caffeinated with half decaffeinated would be a good alternative. You can also start taking more milk (low fat) than coffee, or brew your cups a little less, so they don't have as much caffeine. Focus on slowly replacing the caffeine with other healthier alternatives.

The same goes for your daily pop/soda. Replace your coke with water.

One major key is avoiding caffeine in the afternoon. This is the time of day that has the biggest impact on your sleep. To decrease tiredness you need to improve your quality of sleep; thus, avoid caffeine in the afternoon, as soon as you can manage it.

These tips may not sound easy, but they are doable, and within a matter of weeks you should have a happier, healthier body—with no withdrawal necessary.

One day, these new habits will be so automatic you would have to work to replace them. The difference is you won't need to, because by then you will see how healthy these habits are for you and especially, for your sleep.

Staying Alert without Caffeine

A lot of us use morning coffee as a pick-me-up. We use caffeine to help us remain alert and awake when our bodies don't want to be, because of poor quality sleep. What are some healthier alertness-increasing alternatives?

Exercise is the best alternative. This is because it is very good for your health, your sleep, and most of all it helps you alter your routine instantly. Instead of going to the coffee shop in the morning, why not stop by the gym or use a bedroom floor? The key is to work out and replace the caffeine in your morning routine.

Exercising releases endorphins, a hormone associated with good moods. While getting up to work out may not initially sound like a ton of fun, you'd be surprised at how good it makes your body feel. This is on top of the added health benefits you would get by simply exercising, instead of drinking.

So, what kind of exercise should you do?
You can exercise in any way, from stretching to going for a run; it all depends on your desires and where you are. The ideal morning middle-ground seems to be taking a short walk, but at lunch time you may only have time for some quick stretches, instead of that pop/soda.

Whatever exercise you decide to do, you should already feel happier knowing you have set your body up for a better day, and more importantly, a better night's sleep.

Smoking and Tiredness

Smoking is noticeably bad for your health. It doesn't take a rocket scientist to tell you, the packages even come with pictures. However, did the package warn you that smoking can also contribute to lower quality sleep?

Nicotine increases alertness levels. Since most smokers get their last "fix" before bedtime, they attempt to sleep while totally alert. This can be both frustrating and discouraging for the person trying to sleep. Additionally, middle-of-the-night cravings can wake you, whether you get up to smoke or not, so your quality of sleep is disrupted continually.

Research shows that people who smoke (especially younger people) are four times more likely to suffer from sleep problems than their non-smoking counterparts and spend less time in restful sleep. There are other studies available documenting the detrimental effects of sleep if you are still not convinced, but the truth is smokers do not sleep well.

It is strongly recommended that you kick this habit as soon as possible.

Should you decide to pursue this avenue, there are a myriad of products and programs available to help you quit smoking. It is important to note that these products work for different groups; what works for one person may not work for another and that is okay. There's no sugar-coating this, quitting smoking sucks.

Nicotine is specifically designed to stimulate reactions (and addiction) in your body. It stimulates the hormone adrenaline, which is our old alertness buddy, but it also messes with your system, in excessive amounts.

Forcing your body's energy levels to go through ups and downs throughout the day is not good, regardless of how you are doing it. Nicotine can be especially dangerous, given the other significant health risks to your body.

Nicotine is associated with damage to the respiratory system and cancer.

Benefits of Giving up Smoking

The benefits of giving up smoking are numerous and in some areas, immediate. The following is a non-comprehensive list of the benefits of quitting:

- Improve your breathing abilities
- Enjoy the taste of food with increased enthusiasm
- Healthier look to skin and teeth
- No longer putting friends or family at risk, through second-hand smoke
- Increased alertness

Long term benefits
- Decreased risk to pregnancy and improved fertility levels
- Chances of getting cancer decrease and will eventually be the same as a non-smoker

Quitting Smoking

So, you've decided to quit. You've probably already figured out there's a hard road is ahead. The best thing to do is quit and stay away from it, but this can be easier said than done. The following are some tips to ease the pain and ensure your success.

The first tip is to make a plan. Choose a specific day and *stick to that day*. It doesn't have to be this instant, but when you quit it has to be completely, and that means you need to have whatever you need to quit, ready.

Let your friends know that you're quitting. This serves two different purposes. First, it creates a pride issue for you, so if you fail, you fail more than just yourself and you know it. Second, it lets people know you do not want that cigarette, which encourages support.

Another tip is to set up a system, so the money you would have spent on cigarettes goes to rewarding you. Set it aside in a specific account, so you can see the exact amount you have saved.

One thing that helps is outlining how quitting benefits you. Carry your list with you. Let it remind you why you have quit and why success is so important to you.

An absolutely critical tip is to get rid of all your smoking paraphernalia, to prevent yourself from being reminded of smoking on a daily basis.

The final recommendation is you call yourself a non-smoker. Get used to the idea of being a non-smoker. Make sure you are focused on being in non-smoking areas. Find support via friends, fellow quitters, or support groups.

Acknowledge that this journey will be difficult, but you can make it if you go carefully. You will have cravings, you will want to give up quitting, but you can (and should) plan for these things.

Feel free to try new products and groups until you find one that works for you.

Nicotine Replacement Therapy

Nicotine replacement therapy will be a middle step between cigarettes and quitting.

You will still have some nicotine in the system, but the better you get at using smoking aids, the less of this you will need. It's worth it, because although it still provides you with some nicotine, you will not be taking in other types of toxins that cigarettes contain.

If you prefer to avoid over-the-counter medications, you can seek help from a general practitioner (doctor), for a possible prescription or advice on natural methods (like hypnotism or acupuncture).

There are several varieties of nicotine replacement therapy. Here are some examples:
- Microtabs – dissolve under the tongue
- Nicotine patches or chewing gum
  - Patches come in differing strengths, depending on your needs
- Inhalers – this includes plastic cigarettes
- Nasal sprays - quick-acting for those immediate cravings
- Lozenges – Sucked slowly

Alcohol

To say alcohol is a commonly used substance would be the understatement of the year. While levels of consumption vary from area to area, one common factor, in nearly all cultures, is that it plays a role.

In North America, drinking is primarily social, with an end emphasis placed on intoxication. Intoxication, or "being drunk", can occur from any kind of alcohol, and the reaction itself varies from person to person and situation to situation. What does this mean? You're less likely to get drunk if you're heavier and have eaten a hefty meal first, than if you're petite and haven't eaten all day before you drink. The effects also rely on things like time of day or mood.

For our purposes, alcohol consumption will come in two forms: moderate/healthy and excessive. Excessive drinking leads to a host of problems, because alcohol comes into contact with every organ in the body. Moderate drinking, however, has been linked with (albeit controversial) health benefits—including relaxation. However, any amount of drinking will slow your reaction time.

It is worth noting a lot of people find that "beer makes them sleepy" and they assume that drinking helps them get a good, long sleep. This couldn't be further from the truth, as will be shown.

Now, I'm not going to say you *have* to give up alcohol. Many people point to the unrealistic ideal of letting go of any alcohol consumption as impossible. However, I will lay out options for the person who has chosen to moderately consume it and the person who has chosen to quit it.

The Truth about Sleepiness and Alcohol

The issue with alcohol has nothing to do with getting to sleep—alcohol can indeed help with that, but it does impact the quality of sleep. Alcohol acts as a depressant and often induces tiredness in the short term, but falling asleep doesn't mean you're sleeping well.

Research seems to show that alcohol-induced slumber is far less deep and restful than other sleep. You guessed it: it's that pesky stage five again. People who are drunk spend significantly more time in the earlier stages of sleep, leaving less time for the later stages, which results in exhaustion the next morning.

This effect even takes place when drinking in the afternoon! If you don't believe it, look it up for yourself. Google "alcohol and sleep" and see what comes up.

Another concrete problem with alcohol consumption and sleep is alcohol dehydrates your body. We already mentioned what dehydration does to the sleep cycle, but in brief summary: it keeps you in lighter sleep and keeps a constant fatigue over you.

After finding all this out, if you are looking to cut back on alcohol, or cut it out of your life completely, the next sections are for you.

Cutting Back on Alcohol

The recommended limitations for alcohol consumption are 14 units a week for women and 21 units a week for men (1 unit = spirits, 1.5 = half pint lager or glass of wine).

Don't panic, you can reduce your alcohol intake.

First tip: Stick to smaller alcoholic portions. It may seem more financially responsible to go with the bigger wine glass, but your body will not be thanking you for it later. Furthermore, we finish drinks at the same speed, regardless of size, so the chances of intoxication (and thus, sleep disturbance) increase dramatically.

If you're struggling with the thought of "what will I drink all night?" consider starting with a lighter drink (such as lemonade, a spritzer, or water) for the night. The more light drinks you have, the less big glasses of low quality sleep—I mean alcohol—you will consume.

As with everything else in this guide, a key tip for cutting back on alcohol can be found with water. Water will help your body counteract the negative effects of alcohol, including dehydration.

Finally, don't go out every night. At most, you should go out five nights, and that is the absolute maximum; the fewer nights you spend drinking, the better off your body will be.

If you think none of this sounds remotely possible, you may want to consider the possibility that you have a serious problem with alcohol. If you do have a problem with alcohol **you must seek professional help.** Withdrawal from alcohol addiction can be one of the worst types of withdrawal and you will need help if you are having a serious addiction problem.

Exercise as an Energy Booster

Be prepared, this section ruins a pretty harsh myth. Once you stop thinking it, you'll be shocked at the life changes you'll be inclined to make. Ready? Okay. Exercise does not exhaust you. Exercise actually energizes your body and ultimately, helps you sleep better.

So, when you're saying you're too tired to exercise, what you're actually saying is "I'm too tired to get energy". Sounds crazy, right?

The body uses Adenosine Triphosphate (ATP) for energy consumption. The first source of this is in your diet, specifically glucose. The next source of it is your aerobic system, which burns fat and produces energy. The end result: The more aerobics you engage in, the more awake you will feel.

This is related to how the body adapts. Your body is designed to work best for you. So, if you require a lot of ATP, your body will produce it. If your general heart rate requires your metabolism to run at a faster rate, it will do its best.

Low-Intensity Exercise Reduces Fatigue Symptoms by 65 Percent, Study Finds

This is an example of a study that showcases the efficacy and efficiency of exercising for energy. You don't have to run a marathon or spend all week at the gym, you have to exercise regularly enough that your body knows you need it.

So, get that heart rate up, for 30 minutes of your everyday life. By adding regular exercise to your daily routine, you will find a great reduction in tiredness.

A summary of the science, if it had to be summed up in one line, would be something as follows: the more inactive you are, the less energy you'll have. This is because the body generates energy based on need. If your body only has to lie down all day, it will not be likely at all to energize you for a marathon. That would be inefficient.

Getting Started: A New Routine

One note I will make, before outlining tips on exercising, is if you have not exercised in a long period of time, you may wish to consult your physician before beginning a new routine. This is because your doctor can assess your personal factors, to warn you of any potentially risky exercises for you, and can even point out suitable ones, in some cases.

Medical professionals are also the experts on warning signs, and they can—and will—educate you enough, so you step off that treadmill before you collapse. Remember, we are trying to help you sleep better, not give you a breakdown.

That warning aside, it's time for tips on starting and maintaining an exercise routine.

Developing a routine for you means it has to be a routine that you want to do. Much like the lesson for making your morning fun from earlier, you should pick an exercise routine you can look forward to. Exercise can stress the body, so it helps if you like the type of exercise you're doing.

The next thing I have to say is be sure to be realistic. Again, this guide is not to help you break your body down, it's to help you build yourself up. You can't build anything if you're collapsed and on bed-rest to recover from over-exertion. If you have a hefty fitness goal, consult professionals on the steps you need to take to get there.

There is nobody to stop you from starting small and working your way up to a goal, but don't start at a level that's going to kill you.

Experts recommend doing at least 30 minutes of exercise per day, either by adding time together or doing it all at once.

Squeezing exercise in
For the busy person who feels they have no time, let's consider some exercises you can easily work into your day.

- Go for a walk – whether to the store or around the block, walking is a great form of exercise
- Dance it out – when your favourite song hits the radio and all you want to do is belt it out and dance, do so!
- Take the stairs
- Vacuum to the best of your ability – get down on that floor and reach those edges you normally skip; this is a great practical way to exercise.
- Garden – gardening is a very visually rewarding form of exercise. There are a lot of chores associated with plants (weeding, mowing lawn, raking, etc) that can help you maintain a good fitness level.

We can all do with a little more exercise and these tips help you to fit that in.

Reaching a Bigger Fitness Goal

So, you want to run a marathon, huh? That's great. There's nothing that says doing this is impossible, but it may be currently out of your reach. Let's talk about ways to gradually work up to that 5k.

The reason you want to ease your body into it is because the body is quite vindictive. If you force it to over exert itself, it will retain damage that can cause long term pain, discouragement, and giving up on goals.

By taking the safe alternative of gradually working up to your goal, you are giving the body time to get used to what you want and help you work for it.

Now, what do you do? Pick a program. Base it on your end goal and (more importantly) your current fitness position. You may not be able to run a marathon, but you can walk a few miles, so start with that.

Once you pick a program, *stick with it*. I cannot emphasize this enough. If you miss a day, repeat the exercise on your day off. You need to get three 20 - 30 minute workout sessions in per week, to increase your fitness level.

Let's look at an example of a 5K running plan.

Guidelines
- Make sure you have the appropriate equipment before attempting anything like this. Unsuitable gear is a recipe for disaster.
- Warm up before you do anything! Perhaps a brisk 5 minute walk will help? If you aren't stretching properly, you will get hurt.

-Try to get these sessions in 3 times per week.

Week 1)
    Warm-ups: Take a brisk 5 minute walk.
    The cycle: Run for a minute, walk for 2 minutes, repeat.
    For how long: 20 minutes
    Extra for the week: Take a brisk 30 minute walk.

Week 2)
    Warm-ups: Take a brisk 5 minute walk.
    The cycle: Run for 2 minutes, walk for a minute, repeat.
    For how long: 25 minutes
    Extra for the week: Take a brisk 30 minute walk.

Week 3)
    Warm-ups: Take a brisk 5 minute walk.
    The cycle: Run for 5 minutes, walk for a minute, repeat.
    For how long: 30 minutes
    Extra for the week: Take a brisk 30 minute walk.

Week 4)
    Warm-ups: Take a brisk 5 minute walk.
    The cycle: Run for 8 minutes, walk for a minute, repeat.
    For how long: 30 minutes
    Extra for the week: Take a brisk 30 minute walk.

Week 5)
    Warm-ups: Take a brisk 5 minute walk.
    The cycle: Run for 10 minutes, walk for 2 minutes, run for 8 minutes, walk for 2, run for 6, walk for 2.
    Extra for the week: Take a brisk 30 minute walk.

Week 6)
  Warm-ups: Take a brisk 5 minute walk.
  The cycle: Run for 12 minutes, walk for 2 minutes, run for 12 minutes, walk for 2 minutes, run for 6 minutes.
  Extra for the week: Take a brisk 30 minute walk.

Week 7)
  Warm-ups: Take a brisk 5 minute walk.
  The cycle: Run for 14 minutes, walk for 2 minutes, run for 12.
  Extra for the week: Take a brisk 30 minute walk.

Week 8)
  (This one is only twice per week.)

  Warm-ups: Take a brisk 5 minute walk.
  The cycle: Run for 14 minutes, walk for 2 minutes, run for 14.
  Extra for the week: Take a brisk 30 minute walk.

To understand how this works, look back at what you're doing in week one and compare it directly to week eight. You have started an extra run and are exercising 30 minutes instead of 20, on top of your normal walk!

Maintaining Your Active Lifestyle

Now, you've reviewed ways to add physical activity to your life. Let's talk about how to keep it in your life. Exercise won't do you long-term good if you quit. A lot of people find starting the plan easy, but sticking to it difficult. The following are some tips to help keep you on track.

- Workout with a friend
  This friend must be someone you trust to be honest with you and keep you on task. That being said, find the right buddy and working out is a breeze! Quality time with health benefits? Sign me up!

- Make goals
  You're far more likely to stick to exercising if it helps you with something even if that goal is to not be tired anymore. To make that happen, you must stick to certain tasks.

- Keep an exercise journal
  This includes what you did, how you did it, and the effects. You can also use this journal to record your target goal for that time and track how well you're doing. Tracking improvements helps motivate us in spades.

- Variety is the spice of life
  Make sure that as you become fit, your workout still challenges you. This will maximize your benefits and keep you interested in working out.

- Make exercise part of your routine
  By making sure exercise is part of your daily routine, you will make yourself feel like something is missing when you don't work out. This also helps eradicate the "no time" excuse, because you've made time for it regularly.

Setting Yourself up for a Good Night's Sleep

All we've talked about works to set you up for a good night's sleep, but what about the way you've set up the room you sleep in?

Our brain is very sensitive throughout the night. It keeps waiting for us to demand its immediate use and is always prepared to wake us, if it perceives the need. The problem is this sensitivity can be impacted by a smell, a light, a noise, even simple bodily discomfort.

Warning: Even if the brain doesn't fully wake you up, it does not mean it was not disturbed or brought you back to lighter stages of sleep.

Every time we wake up, our sleep cycle is interrupted and starts over. This is bad for the quality of our sleep. I'm now going to lay out some tips that will help you set up your room for a good night's sleep.

First off, recognize that you can't control everything. It's a fact. Sometimes there's noise and there's no point getting angry at the source of it. This guide focuses on the things that you *can* control and how to specifically alter them.

Air

It seems like air is a good place to begin. Try to remember back to a hot, stuffy attic you tried to sleep in, as a child (likely at grandma's house). You probably weren't very comfortable, were you? Discomfort equals sleep disruption (I'll say it again and again).

So what do you do?

Provide a humidifier for your bedroom. This prevents the air from getting dry.

Colour
Try to pick a colour that you identify as being peaceful for your bedroom. This can be blue, green, purple, or other muted tones. The important thing is that it makes you feel calm.

Temperature
Being uncomfortably warm or uncomfortably cold can cause discomfort. We've learned time and time again by this point, discomfort means disruptions to sleep. So, what do you want to do? Avoid uncomfortable temperatures.

General recommendations for what "room temperature" is tend to fall in the 20 – 22 degrees Celsius (68 – 72 Fahrenheit) range. This can vary, depending on the individual, so as with many of these tips, you should experiment and jot down notes on how different temperatures serve you, until you find your ideal.

Obviously, most of this control will take place at your thermostat, but it can be as simple as changing your bedding with the seasons. You need a warmer comforter in December than in May, so make sure you're providing yourself with one.

Light
Our melatonin levels respond negatively to light; the more light there is, the less melatonin we have, and the less tired you are. The good news is the opposite

is true as well: when it is dark, we become progressively more tired.

So, what should you do in your bedroom? Keep it as dark as possible at night, to help your body regulate melatonin levels. Have curtains (or blinds, drapes, etc) cover the windows to block out night light.

Consider purchasing an eye mask if you cannot eliminate all of the light in your room.

By combining the effects of an eye mask and good window curtains/covers, even one who sleeps throughout the day and wakes at night can have a healthy sleep life. These methods are not all that difficult or complicated to implement, and you'll see the results from your body to thank you for it.

Sound
Sound is a good example of an interference that can disrupt your sleep, without fully waking you. Ever hear the doorbell in your dream and find out later your friend was waiting for you? This is because the brain filtered the sound into your mind. This results in—you guessed it—less REM sleep and deep sleep, in general.

The first tip is to make sure your windows are as insulated as they can be. This is a move that must either be made early, or compensated for with window coverings.

There are also machines that you can purchase that provide solid "white noise" (irrelevant background sound) that blocks out/covers other noises. Some people find particular soothing noises and buy CDs of them.

The next idea for you to consider is trying earplugs. Earplugs can be bought fairly cheap and there are tons available. You should continue trying products until you find the right one for you—the one that blocks out noise. The bottom line is you are looking for what can help you sleep well each night and you should not be hearing noise.

There is some good news in this regard, in that our brains are able to filter out normal, non-alarming sounds with little difficulty. You don't typically wake up to a drawer opening, but you probably will to a siren or the radio.

This is great, because there's no way we can absolutely keep all noise out of our rooms. In fact, we shouldn't want to (we're not used to the quiet, but we can use the tips above to reduce disturbances, while trying to rest.

Pajamas
The main thing we will say about your clothing is make it loose and comfortable. Give your body room to move and breathe throughout the night. That is the main consideration. Your comfort is important to your sleep quality, whether you're comfiest in cotton or in wool.

The only other thing to say about this is making sure you are staying appropriately warm or cool, depending on the season, can be part of temperature regulation.

Bedding
Make sure your bedding is adequately comfortable and enables your temperature regulation. Having multiple layers is a great idea, because it enables you to

discard unnecessary layers on hot nights, or add on extra for those cold winter mornings.

A note: it can be tempting to go blanket free, but this is an error in judgement. When we are warm, we sweat, which messes with our brain, which can disrupt our sleep. Covering with a thin blanket should be sufficient to keep you from sweating and keep your temperature at an appropriate level.

Also, make sure that you have adequate pillows and mattresses backing your linens. If you don't have adequate sleeping provisions, you won't sleep well. This means replacing old mattresses and pillows!

Pillows come in a variety of materials. You can choose from down filling to memory foam; the choice can be intimidating, given the number of options. Keep in mind the purpose of the pillow: it support your head and neck. This also relates to when pillows get old. When pillows are flat, they are no longer adequately supporting your head, which can cause tension. Get rid of that pillow, and buy a new one, perhaps while you're out buying a new mattress.

Mattresses have a life of approximately ten years. It is worth spending money to replace old mattresses with new ones. It is also important to think about the material you are sleeping on, whether memory foam or box-spring. Remember, this is your body's health, is it really a good time to go cheap? No.

Invest in yourself and make sure you have the right bedding materials.

Buying the Right Mattress for You

The primary point I can make to you about purchasing a mattress is to try it out. This does not mean going to sleep for hours and hours, but it does mean climbing onto a bed you are considering purchasing. Lay down in your normal position. It feels embarrassing, but taking care of your body is worth it, and salespeople will reassure you, they see it all the time.

While you're lying down, take time to ask the salesperson some questions. How long should this mattress last? Is there a warranty? What does it cover? What is this fabric good for?

These tips are all critical to setting your bed up for the right kind of sleep.

Power Naps

We've talked a lot about how to improve your night time sleep, but what about naps? Power naps are short periods of sleep that are meant to get you back on your feet and ready to finish the day. Thomas Edison was an advocate of the power nap. Claims surrounding his history range wildly, but it seems as though he would sleep only a short amount at night and take a two hour nap throughout the day, to supplement his energy levels. (This is similar to the polyphasic sleep schedule we will talk about later.)

Naps can be effective, but only if understood and used correctly. Research is divided on the exact effects of napping, but it has repeatedly pointed to the positive alertness effects of napping, depending on the person. Humorously enough, some studies have shown that naps are most effective when taken with a cup of coffee. Given the short length of power naps, it seems the caffeine provides an extra kick.

Another study showed that specifically 20-minute-long naps could be more beneficial than sleeping late in the morning.

Power napping is recommended in some cases, but only when acting as a supplement, not a replacement, for a good night's sleep.

Obviously, efficient napping is done in such a way to prevent you from coming away with an incomplete sleep cycle; otherwise, how would it help your alertness? Ranges for good napping times go from one to two hours, although generally not less than that. However, it does change from one person to another.

Another obstacle to napping is the full-time job. Most of us don't have time to take an hour off, but 15 minutes could be doable. Part of this will be trial and error, and figuring out what your body needs to function well.

If you want to try napping, keep in mind the following:
- Watch the clock (do not nap longer than two hours or shorter than 15 minutes)
- Experiment to see your ideal length of naptime
- **Do not attempt to replace night time sleep with a nap in the day**

Sleeping Less

Way back in the beginning of this book, we mentioned the possibility of sleeping less. Tina Hagen and Peter Novak's "End Tiredness Program" is an excellent way to do this.

If you have followed along so far, you already know how many cycles of sleep you personally need and how long each of your cycles take. Reducing your amount of time spent in bed can be as simple as cutting back on the number of cycles and allowing the others to optimize themselves, to give yourself the same amount of energy output as before.

You can experiment with this by adjusting your sleep schedule to allow for one less cycle and evaluating how this makes you feel in the days that follow the change. If you are still operating at full efficiency, you can conceivably repeat this process.

Note: Your body will take time to adjust when you play with these cycles, so give yourself a few weeks (wherein you power nap, if necessary) and record how you feel, before making the decision to return to old patterns or keep up with the new one.

Experimenting like this is a perfectly legitimate option when you are careful to monitor yourself.

Feng Shui

Many people believe that feng shui can influence their relaxation levels. Feng shui is an ancient Chinese art that focuses on arranging a room, in a way that promotes relaxation. Although findings on this are mixed, some people claim it works. This could easily be because some feng shui advice aligns perfectly with the practical advice found in this guide already.

An example of this is the removal of distraction. Feng shui requires all electronic forms of entertainment be removed from the. This advice lines up with the thought of preparing your bedroom for sleep and not for other activities of day.

Other examples in feng shui that appear in practical advice involve lighting and air. You should use candles instead of lights and prevent stale air from circulating by letting air into your room.

Feng shui also suggests that you regulate the art you choose to hang, the position of your bed, and the use of mirrors. Let's use the example of the position of the bed: feng shui dictates that the bed be approachable from both sides, to allow the total flow of energy throughout the night. Similarly, the mirror should NOT face the bed, to avoid messing with the flow of energy.

If you are interested in the rules of feng shui, feel free to look into them. These principles seem effective for some at least, so if you want to try it, feel free.

Alternative Holistic Therapies

We've already discussed many of the unhealthy alternatives to a good night's sleep (energy drinks, caffeine, and so on). There have been steps provided, so that you can achieve a better night's sleep, but what if you need something different? We will now consider alternative therapies.

Aromatherapy

Aromatherapy uses essential oils to affect the mind. There are professional aroma therapists and amateur home aromatherapy kits. You can decide which is right for you.

The general recommendation is that you use aromatherapy in connection with your nightly bath, putting a few drops of sleep-inducing scents into the water, before climbing into bed.

Herbalism

There are many popular herbal aids for sleep, from passionflower to valerian. Valerian seems to be a popular remedy, so we shall consider it here.

Valerian is typically taken once a night, for a few weeks, to induce sleepiness. This herb is typically found in capsule supplements or tea drinks.

Teas are quite popular for distribution of herbal remedies; even the warmth of the drink itself can make you drowsy. They also make excellent replacements for those bad dietary habits you need to break.

There are countless alternative therapies if you are interested and it is absolutely fine to look into them. However, be sure you get advice from someone who knows what they are doing and you will be well on your way to preparing yourself for a good night's sleep.

Polyphasic Sleep

Some people trying to make the most out of bedtime have start a polyphasic sleep pattern. A polyphasic sleep pattern is when you sleep repeatedly throughout the day, but never all at once (this is monophasic).

The research has been quite mixed on this. Critics claim that this can easily lead to sleep deprivation, causing ultimately more damage than it's worth. Critics are quite bleak about what this can do. However, people who are doing it claim that it increases your alertness levels and healthiness.

Personal accounts, available online, tend to be quite positive of the shift (although it is difficult to get the body to adjust, initially). Interestingly enough, not many people seem to permanently make the switch; several of those who rave about it one day revert to monophasic sleep cycles the next. This type of sleep cycle could be more conducive to a hectic work schedule, or certain periods of life, rather than a life-long method of sleeping.

Part of the problem with this research conflict could also be that there is a variety of polyphasic sleep programs.

It is a personal choice, so whatever you decide, make sure you are doing your research and remaining safe!

Reflexology and Other Relaxation Techniques

Reflexology focuses on massage techniques to medically induce relaxation. It tends to focus on the hands, feet, and ears, but benefits far more than that, according to its claims.

Reflexology works by focusing on relaxation and balance in its techniques. The touch is used to help inspire the body to work on itself as you rest, making it a nicely complementary technique for any of the tips here.

It has quite the modern appeal. You can learn to turn yourself off for sleepiness, or have your partner help you drift off to sleep. There are a lot of positive reports reviewing reflexology, but only from those who take it seriously.

Many look at reflexology and assume it's an excuse to get a massage from their partners. Reflexologists would certainly reject this, as the goal of reflexology is much higher than that. The goal of reflexology is to manipulate certain parts of the body, to affect the body as a whole.

Reiki

Reiki (universal energy) is a spiritually-oriented form of therapy. It began in Japan, and is meant to be a non-manipulative treatment. The process is as follows: a therapist (or yourself) runs their hands over the body, drawing in energy and relaxation. It claims to help tiredness, specifically by relaxing the body and thus, relaxing the mind.

While research does not specifically confirm or deny the claims of Reiki, the ultimate bottom line to quality sleep is being tired – and being relaxed enough to get there.

If you do decide that you'd like to try an alternative form of therapy (be it reflexology or feng shui), make sure you do your research to get valid advice and you implement that advice. It means nothing for you to attempt to discredit a technique, without actually having tried it.

Conclusions

Going without sleep has caused death in laboratory animals and had extremely damaging health effects to human beings, as well. From headaches to drowsiness, all the way to increasing irritability, a bad night's sleep is not something to shrug off.

This guide has provided you with the tips and information to improve your sleep, in several different ways. Obviously; most people will not take on every single piece of advice given here, but that's fine; this is a guide to a massive field of research and cultural ideas.

The most important key is sleeping needs to be taken seriously. You need to work out your personal needs and ensure that you are getting them. Feel free to move freely between this book's chapters. From feng shui to exercising, there is a lot in here.

It is our sincerest hope that you found this entire report helpful and will start your own sleep journal, too! I personally challenge you to test the effects for yourself.

Subscribe to our newsletter for strategies to better
health, naturally!
www.naturesnaturalhealth.com/join